DEDICATION

This book is dedicated to Grace-Kelly Jacqueline Fender and my mother Martine Calache, CCH, RsHOM, DiHom, FHom. Without both of you I would not be here.

DISCLAIMER

This homeopathic materia medica and repertory set is provided for information purposes only, with no guarantee of accuracy. It is not intended as a substitute for medical advice, nor as a claim for the effectiveness of homeopathic remedies in treating any of the symptoms mentioned in these books. If the symptoms persist, seek professional medical advice. Minor symptoms can often be a sign of a more serious underlying condition.

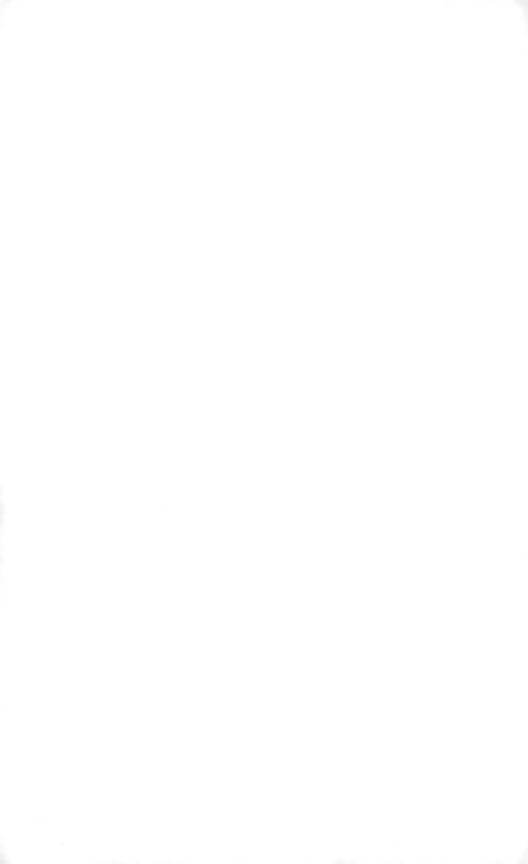

Table of Contents

About The Author

Liza Calache

Liza is a 3rd generation homeopath with formal education beginning at just 12 years old. Sitting amongst medical professionals, Liza took advantage of every learning opportunity presented to her. While studying under world-renowned homeopath and professor, Luc De Schepper, MD, Liza acquired a vast amount of knowledge that would set the stage for further homeopathic prospects. Upon completion of her formal education, which lasted 15 years, she began teaching and practicing alongside her mother, Martine Calache, CCH, DiHOM, RsHOM, FHom. While being able to practice and teach, Liza has also acquired a bachelor of science in Chemistry and was certified by the state of New Jersey as a secondary education teacher. She applied her knowledge of chemistry, homeopathy and education together and was able to write her own chemistry text book for high school students. During her time as a high school teacher, she was nominated for teacher of the year for her unique ability to work with disadvantaged students with low learning abilities and transform how they learn. In 2013, Liza was blessed with a baby girl that would change her life. Liza continues to teach and practice Homeopathy with her mother in the school they named, First Class Homeopathy. She is in her final steps in completing her board certification with The Council of Homeopathic Certification.

HOW TO USE THIS SET OF BOOKS

These books are intended to be used as a quick and simple reference guide to finding the most appropriate homeopathic remedy based upon the symptoms of the child. It is a compilation of facts gathered from several well-known authors and trusted sources in homeopathy. Straight to the point, with all the facts you need to get the right remedy fast, and all in one book!

Homeopathy works by balancing the person's immune system so that it can heal itself of whatever ailment it is battling. Since homeopathy is a holistic form of alternative medicine, it is based on the symptoms of the whole body: mental, emotional and physical. To find the appropriate remedy, it is VITAL that ALL or AS MANY AS POSSIBLE symptoms are noted. The remedy that matches the symptoms is the best one to give. This is easier to do with an adult who can effectively communicate their symptoms to you. The challenge comes with a child and even more so with an infant who cannot speak yet. In these cases, the power of OBSERVATIONS becomes extremely useful. The key is to be as descriptive as possible with noting the symptoms. For example, your child might tell you, "My throat hurts." If I were to research "sore throat" in the books, I would find at least 50 remedies! Ask your child some questions to get a more descriptive answer. Here are some questions to help you out:

Where does it hurt? Is it your whole throat, or does one side hurt more than the other? Would it make it better if you drank some hot milk or any kind of hot beverage? Does it feel burning? Does it hurt when you swallow?

Obviously this becomes a challenge with an infant. So observe when the baby is eating, does she pull away from bottle or breast? Do they take little sips, pause, and resume? Are they scratching the outside of their throat?

Now that you have your description, it's time to look up the main symptom. Let's use sore throat as our example. When you find sore throat, you will see all the possible remedies for this ailment. Now that you have your description, all you have to do is match the remedy that most looks like your child's description. The first column tells you the name of the remedy with its common abbreviation. The second column tells you how that remedy is different from the other remedies in that section. You may find that there could be two or three remedies that could fit your

1

description. In this case, the third column was added. The third column tells you how to distinguish that remedy from other close matches by listing the most common ailments that remedy has.   If a column field is left blank, it is intentional as there is no evidence of further differentiation.

A Few Words About Potencies

Now that you have found the remedy you will give, what strength do you give the remedy and how do you give it? There are several ways to do this, but I will show you the most updated way that is absorbed into the body most efficiently. To do this it is important to understand what the different "potencies" or strengths are available and in which events they are most commonly used.

6C
30C
200C
1000C or 1M
10000C or 10M
100000C or 100M or CM

When you purchase a homeopathic remedy, on the tube should have the name of the remedy and a number and a letter after it. This number and letter indicate the potency or strength that the remedy was made in. Each potency has a different purpose. The rule of thumb in classical homeopathic prescribing is to take into account the persons sensitivity. We do not want make the person feel any worse than they already do. While homeopathy has no side-effects, it is possible to "aggravate" the persons symptoms. What this means is that you have chosen the correct remedy for their symptoms, but the potency was too strong for their immune system to handle. In this case, their symptoms are worsened until the aggravation wears off. In order to prevent aggravations, do not give a potency that is too high. For children, it is best that 6C or 30C is given for everyday ailments such as cold, flu, teething, etc. When there is an emergency, the most common potencies used are 200C and 1M. Very rarely would anyone use 10M or CM potencies. As homeopaths, we always have two choices for potencies because of the sensitivities of the patient. If we know the person is sensitive, we start with the lower potency. If after giving the remedy we notice that it does not work, the next step is to increase the potency as it might have been too low. If again it does not work, it probably is safe to say you did not choose the correct remedy. How long do you wait to determine if you need to change potency or change remedy? Usually by 3-4 doses if there is no response, make the necessary changes.

Now that you know which potencies to use, how do you administer the remedy? As Hahnemann (founder of homeopathy) stated in his last edition of his manual (Organon of Homeopathy 5th & 6th edition), for acute situations the protocol is as follows:

2 pellets of the remedy in a 4 ounce bottle. Mix around. Take 1 teaspoon from bottle. Repeat as necessary until symptoms disappear. With each time the remedy is repeated, it is important to succuss the bottle each time BEFORE you take it.

What are succussions?

A Succussion is a forceful hitting on the bottom of the bottle, usually with one's palm.

What is the purpose of succussions?

I will try to explain this as simple as possible, and this is where some chemistry comes in. Every object contains energy. There are two main categories of energies that exist: kinetic and potential. Kinetic is energy of motion and potential is stored energy or energy of its position. If something is not moving or at rest, it has potential energy until it is in motion, which will then change to kinetic energy. This is exactly what we want to do with the remedy. Each time we take the remedy, we want to "activate" the molecules and make sure they are "moving around" so we hit the bottom of the bottle; succussions. Each time the bottle is succussed, the remedy gets stronger. How is that possible? This is how the remedies were originally made when you bought them in the little tubes. Homeopathic remedies are not made solely on dilutions.

How are homeopathic remedies made from the original substance?

One drop of the substance is needed and either 9 or 99 drops of alcohol is added. 9 drops to make an "X" potency, and 99 drops to make a "C" potency scale. For our purposes, we are using the "C" scale. So 99 drops of alcohol is added to the 1 drop of the plant extract, making it 100 drops…that's where the "C" comes from (from the latin for 100). If you were to stop here, this would just be a dilution…not a homeopathic remedy. To make it a remedy, it has been succussed 100 times. Now you will have a 1C remedy. To get to desired number, repeat the process. Thankfully, there is no need to make these remedies since there are several companies that have already done that for us. This information is useful if you were in the jungle and saw a plant of the remedy and decided to make a remedy there because you forgot your kit!

How many succussions do you do before you take the remedy?

You can do anywhere from 2-8 succussions but remember, this makes the remedy stronger each time it is done. Therefore, remember that the person's sensitivity is important here. We do not want to aggravate. If they are sensitive, a good rule is 2-4, if they are not they can probably handle 6-8.

JAUNDICE

REMEDIES:

Chelidonium, China, Natrum Sulph., Lycopodium

Remedy	Symptom Differentiation	Keynote Differentiation
Chel	Yellow face, worse on nose and cheeks	This remedy has an affinity for the liver. Constant pain under right scapula, feels everything is great effort, better from eating dinner and pressure, worse from motion/touch/change of weather/early morning
Chin	Unhealthy yellow or pale brown face	This remedy is known for ringing and buzzing in ears, hypersensitivity of senses, hypotension, bitter taste in mouth, gas, worse from drafts/slight pressure/every other day/beer/milk/fruit, better from heat and strong pressure, no appetite, loss of vital fluids, pulsating headaches, hemorrhages
Nat Sulph	Yellow looking eyes	This remedy has an affinity for digestive, respiratory and nervous system, with effects on the joints and skin, worse from cold and humidity, intense thirst especially for cold drinks, watery stool that squirt out especially in the morning, bronchitis, asthma in children, holds chest when coughing
Lyc	Grayish-yellow color of face with blue circles around eyes	This remedy has an affinity for liver and digestion, kidneys and genitals, mucus and skin, and nervous system. Worse between 4-8pm, worse with heat, better with cool air, craving for sweets and oysters, ravenous appetite, flatulence, bloating after meals, doesn't like

		tight clothes on waist, abdomen is distended, red face after eating, migraine from poor digestion, bedwetting, nose stuffy with crusty mucus especially at night, sleep with mouth open, runny nose during day, anorexia in children

LACTOSE INTOLERANCE

REMEDIES:

Aethusa, Calcarea Carb., Calcarea Phos., Calcarea Silicatum, Kali Iodatum, Natrum Carb., Sepia, Silica, Tuberculinum

Remedy	Symptom Differentiation	Keynote Differentiation
Aeth	Intolerant to mother's milk, diarrhea	This remedy has an affinity for the digestive and nervous system. Profuse diarrhea and severe vomiting, cannot tolerate milk, total exhaustion, no thirst, consequences of over-feeding child, lack of concentration in children
Calc Carb	Diarrhea from milk	Any Calcarea remedy has an affinity for bones, lymph nodes, circulation and polyps. They sweat profusely on head, babies teethe late, walk slow and are lazy, large appetite, remember the four F's: fat, fair skin, fainting, and fearful. If Ruta and Rhus Tox have stopped working, this remedy can be thought of. For chronic indications of pulsatilla
Calc Phos	Intolerant to mother's milk	This remedy has an affinity for the bones, blood, lymph nodes and works on the nutrition of the body. Teeth are long, narrow and yellow, bones are long and straight, tired and

		nervous, rickets, weight loss, repetitive sore throat/bronchitis/colds
Calc Sil	Intolerant to cold milk	Very sensitive to cold, weakness, emaciation, worse from being over-heated, very thirsty, irritable
Kali Iod	Intolerant to cold milk	This remedy has an affinity for the mucus and lymphatic system. Worse from heat and at night, better from cold temperature/fresh air/moving around, burning/watery/abundant mucus
Nat Carb	Diarrhea from milk	This remedy has an affinity for the nervous and digestive system. Worse from heat/cold/music/mental activity, better from motion, headaches from exposure to sun, diarrhea with urgency to go with yellow stools with orange pulp-like substances
Sep	Intolerant to boiled and room temperature milk, diarrhea from milk	This remedy has an affinity for the circulatory and nervous system. Hormonal imbalance. Sitting or kneeling for long periods causes fainting, worse before storm, better with exercise, feels like abdomen is heavy, flushes of heat in face, craves vinegar, and sour foods, worse 11 am
Sil	Intolerant to mother's milk, diarrhea from milk	This remedy has an affinity for the nervous system and is very malnourished. They are weak and demineralized. Worse cold and humid weather, better with heat, slinters (will push them out), fontanels stay open, perspire on head, abscess remedy, white spots on nails,

		weak nails/hair
Tub	Intolerant to mother's milk	Nervous hypersensitivity, rapid weight loss, extreme sensitivity to cold, slow physical development, very dissatisfied, worse from least exercise/standing/change in weather/stuffy room, better from outside/fresh air/rest/continuous movement, cough at night, craving for cold milk even if they are intolerant of, uncontrollable diarrhea at 5am

LEARNING DISABILITIES/HYPERACTIVITY

REMEDIES:

Arsenicum Album, Cina, Hyoscyamus, Iodum, Stramonium, Tarentula, Veratrum Album

Remedy	Symptom Differentiation	Keynote Differentiation
Ars	Great restlessness, changes places continually	This remedy has an affinity for mucus, kidneys liver, adrenal glands and the nervous system. This remedy can be summed up in three words: weak, restless and cold (temperature-wise). Burning pains, worse 1-3am and from the cold, thirsty for small amounts of cold water, fear of death, food-poisoning
Cina	Ill-humored child, very cross, does not wnt to be touched, desires many things but rejects them when offered	Convulsions beginning on one side of the face, attack stops and begins at the same time, breathing slows down, urine incontinence, do not like to be touched or looked

8

		at, large circles under the eyes, sickly appearance, yawn frequently, grinding of teeth, restless sleep, frequent rubbing of nose and scratching of nostrils, constant hunger that is not easily satiable, pain in belly-button better by lying on abdomen, worse during new moon and full moon, better lying on stomach/abdomen, presence of round worms, teething
Hyos	Nervous agitation, very talkative, foolish behavior	This remedy has an affinity for the nervous system. Laughs at everything, uncovers body, jealous, foolish, attempting to run away, muttering speech, quarrelsome, sobs and cries without waking up, worse at night/after eating/lying down
Iod	Anxiety when quiet, must keep busy	This remedy has an affinity for the thyroid. Rapid metabolism,
Stram	Extremely talkative, laughing/singing/swearing/praying	This remedy has an affinity for the brain and the nervous system. Worse in dark/shinny and bright objects/being alone, better from soft light and being around people, severe and violent convulsions, incoherent talkativeness, hallucinations, nightmares, swollen tongue, doesn't like the sight of liquids, spasmodic

		and suffocative cough, bright red rash
Tarent	Sudden change of moods, must constantly stay busy, extreme restlessness	This remedy has a feeling of constriction. Sensitive to music, must dance when hearing music, dances in patterns, prefers to be alone, vertigo, nymphomania, twitching and jerking of hands and legs, worse from motion/contact/noise, better in open air/music/bright colors/rubbing
Verat Al	Frenzy of excitement, cursing	This remedy has an affinity for the digestive and nervous system. Weakness, collapsing, exhaustion, cold sweats on forehead, coldness all over body, burning inside of body, large amounts of vomiting/diarrhea/ perspiration, worse cold and humid weather, better heat, cholera-like diarrhea

LEARNING DISABILITIES/POOR CONCENTRATION

REMEDIES:

Aethusa, Baryta Carb., Carcinosinum, Medorrhinum, Phosphorus, Helleborus, Nux Vomica, Silica

Remedy	Symptom Differentiation	Keynote Differentiation
Aeth	Lack of concentration while studying	This remedy has an affinity for the digestive and nervous system. Profuse diarrhea and severe vomiting, cannot tolerate milk, total exhaustion, no thirst, consequences of over-feeding child, lack of concentration in

		children
Bar Carb	Lack of concentration while studying	This remedy has an affinity for the mental development, arteries, and lymphatic system. Late development/milestones, shy, worse cold/humid/thinking about problems
Carc	Lack of concentration while studying	This remedy has an affinity for the breasts and the uterus. Indigestion, gas in stomach and stools, rheumatism
Med	Lack of concentration, can't fix attention	This remedy has an affinity for the nervous system. Pains are intolerable, children are dwarfed and stunted in growth, weak memory, cries when speaking, when speaking they lose their train of thought, fear of the dark and someone is behind them
Phos	Lack of concentration while studying, can't fix attention	This remedy is highly sensitive especially to light, noises, and smells. Fear of thunderstorm, worse from cold/storms/left side, better from sleep, craves salt and cold drinks, midnight "snacker" especially around 3 am, #1 morning sickness remedy
Hell	Lack of concentration while studying, slow in answering, thoughtless	This remedy has an affinity for the senses. Worse from 4-8pm, staring, involuntary sighing, complete unconsciousness, picks at their lips and clothes, sudden screaming and moaning, beats head into pillow and with hands, breath is offensive, grinding teeth
Nux Vom	Lack of concentration while studying	This remedy as an affinity for the nervous and digestive system. Irritable, cold, hypersensitive, angry, worse

		after eating, better with sleep, tongue is yellow/white color, craves spicy and sour food, constipation, sneezing upon waking
Sil	Lack of concentration while studying, can't fix attention	This remedy has an affinity for the nervous system and is very malnourished. They are weak and demineralized. Worse cold and humid weather, better with heat, slinters (will push them out), fontanels stay open, perspire on head, abscess remedy, white spots on nails, weak nails/hair

LEARNING DISABILITIES/SPEECH/READING/MATH MISTAKES

REMEDIES:

Ammonium Carb., Calcarea Carb., China, Crotalus Horr., Hyoscyamus, Lachesis Lycopodium, Natrum Mur., Nux Vomica, Mercurius Sol., Thuja,

Remedy	Symptom Differentiation	Keynote Differentiation
Amm Carb	Mistakes in mathematics/speaking/writing/misplacing words, using wrong words, calls things by wrong name	This remedy has heaviness in all organs. Nosebleeds after washing and eating, congestion at night, mucus is bloody, mouth is dry, enlarged tonsils, heartburn, bleeding hemorrhoids
Calc Carb	Mistakes in speaking/writing/misplacing words/reversing words/differentiating in objects, using wrong words, calls things by wrong name	Any Calcarea remedy has an affinity for bones, lymph nodes, circulation and polyps. They sweat profusely on head, babies teethe late, walk slow and are lazy, large appetite,

		remember the four F's: fat, fair skin, fainting, and fearful. If Ruta and Rhus Tox have stopped working, this remedy can be thought of. For chronic indications of pulsatilla
China	Mistakes in speaking/writing/misplacing words/reverses words, using wrong words, transposing letters	This remedy is known for ringing and buzzing in ears, hypersensitivity of senses, hypotension, bitter taste in mouth, gas, worse from drafts/slight pressure/every other day/beer/milk/fruit, better from heat and strong pressure, no appetite, loss of vital fluids, pulsating headaches, hemorrhages
Crot H	Mistakes in mathematics/speaking/writing/mispl acing words, using wrong words	This remedy has an affinity for the blood. Hemorrhaging, crying, memory is cloudy, impatient, very talkative, vertigo, very sensitive to light, eyes look yellow, blood oozes from ears, blood is black and stringy, throat feels constricted/tight/swoll en/red, right side of body feels paralyzed
Hyos	Mistakes in differentiating objects/reading/speaking/misplacing words, using wrong words	This remedy has an affinity for the nervous system. Laughs at everything, uncovers body, jealous, foolish, attempting to run away,

		muttering speech, quarrelsome, sobs and cries without waking up, worse at night/after eating/lying down
Lach	Mistakes in mathematics/locations/reading/spelling/ speaking/misplacing words/time (always imagines it afternoon)/writing	This remedy has an affinity for the nervous system and blood. Bruising, hemorrhaging, blotchy face, talkative, suspicious, jealous, spiteful, depression, worse from discharges that are delayed or insufficient/being touched/sun/heat/sleeping/tight clothes/left side, better from discharge that finally comes out, insomnia (especially before midnight), dreams of ghosts, dead people, coffins, difficulty swallowing, sinusitis, apnea, hot flushes in head, ulcers, bed sores
Lyc	Mistakes in mathematics/speaking/writing/spelling/misplacing words, using wrong words, adds letters	This remedy has an affinity for liver and digestion, kidneys and genitals, mucus and skin, and nervous system. Worse between 4-8pm, worse with heat, better with cool air, craving for sweets and oysters, ravenous appetite, flatulence, bloating after meals, doesn't like tight clothes on waist, abdomen is distended,

		red face after eating, migraine from poor digestion, bedwetting, nose stuffy with crusty mucus especially at night, sleep with mouth open, runny nose during day, anorexia in children
Nat Mur	Mistakes in locations/speaking/writing/misplacing words, using wrong words	This remedy can be summed up with three words: Malnutrition, dehydrated and weak. Worse being consoled, worse 10am, worse when at the ocean, loss of vital fluids will cause symptoms, discharge is clear and in large quantities, craves salt, eczema in the creases of joints/forehead/edge of scalp, herpetic rashes especially after illness, dry and cracked skin, chapped lips
Nux Vom	Mistakes in mathematics/differentiating objects/locations/speaking/writing/misplacing words, using wrong words	This remedy as an affinity for the nervous and digestive system. Irritable, cold, hypersensitive, angry, worse after eating, better with sleep, tongue is yellow/white color, craves spicy and sour food, constipation, sneezing upon waking
Merc Sol	Mistakes in mathematics/locations/speaking/using wrong words/misplacing words	This remedy has an affinity for the digestive and renal systems with specific action on throat. Foul-smelling

		breath, gums are white/yellow color and ulcers in gums, tooth abscess, sores in mouth, intense thirst, thick tongue, salivate heavily, parotiditis, heavy perspiration especially at night and offensive in odor, ulcers, worse at night, known as "the human thermometer," shivering and goose-bumps
Thuja	Mistakes in mathematics/speaking/using wrong words/writing	This remedy has an affinity for the skin, mucus, and any type of growths appearing inside of body or outside on the skin: warts, moles, acne, seborrhea, cradle cap, hair loss, scalp has white scaly dandruff Worse cold/humid weather/3 am or 3 pm, better with heat, discharges have a moldy smell

LICE

REMEDIES:

Staphysagria

Remedy	Symptom Differentiation	Keynote Differentiation
Staph	Mosquitos and lice prevention and treatment	To prevent, make up remedy and put in a spray bottle. Spray desired areas. This can be used for pets as well. This remedy has an affinity for

		the urinary and genital system as well as the skin. Hypersensitive to emotions, excitable, irritated easily, obsessed about sexual ideas, burning/frequent/dripping urination, eczema with severe itching, styes especially on upper eyelids

MEASELES

REMEDIES:

Aconite, Apis, Belladonna, Bryonia, Euphrasia, Gelsemium, Kali Bich., Pulsatilla, Sulphur

Remedy	Symptom Differentiation	Keynote Differentiation
Acon	Beginning stage of measles, high fever, cough is dry and barking, pink eye, skin is itchy and burns, restlessness, anxiety, fearful, tosses and turns	This remedy has an affinity for the circulatory and nervous system. Worse extreme or sudden cold/extreme heat/night, better with perspiration, rapid pulse, sudden high fever, red skin, intense thirst for large quantities of cold water, restlessness, anxiety, fear of death, croup cough
Apis	Rash doesn't fully develop then disappears, child still feels unwell, skin is itchy, eyes and face are puffy, worse from warmth	This remedy is known for swelling, burning pain, and jealousy. Worse from heat, better from cold, hot dry skin, inflammation
Bell	Beginning stage of measles, sudden onset, high fever, red face, headache is throbbing, drowsy, delirious, insomnia, thirstless	Symptoms usually have sudden and violent onset, local congestion of blood (example face is red), the congested area is usually hot, children usually convulse when they have a fever
Bry	Delayed rash, cough is hard and dry, no mucus, worse from motion, delirious	Very thirsty especially if during a fever, sinuses are very dry (hint to remember: if dry think

17

		"bry"), pressure headaches that usually travel from forehead to occiput, or can start from left eye and move to the back of the head
Euph	Fever and rash, eyes tearing, nose discharge is non-irritating, worse from light, cough during daytime, measles with common cold	This remedy has an affinity for the nose and the eyes. Pink eye, eyes clump together, worse heat/wind/night, better in the dark, measles
Gels	Low grade fever, weak, heavy, thirstless, headache	This remedy is known for fever (low-grade), circulatory and digestive system, paralysis of nerves and respiratory muscles. Trembling, congestion, sleepy, stiffness, depressed state, worse from heat/hot weather/bad news, better from urinating/sweating/movements, thirstless during fever, migraine or congestion headaches, red face
Kali Bich	Nose discharge is ropy and string, eyes are burning and tearing, glands are swollen, ear pain is stitching and moves from ear-head-neck	This remedy has an affinity for mucus and the skin. Worse cold/2-3am/movement/drinking beer, better with heat, pains start and stop suddenly, aphthae in mouth, thirsty for beer, burning pain in stomach, sciatica left side, heel pain, ulcers, headaches from digestive issues
Puls	Mild form of measles, low grade fever, eyes tearing profusely, nose discharge in large amount, cough is dry (night) and loose (day), ear inflammation, mouth is dry, thirstless	This remedy has an affinity for the venous system and mucus. Changeable behavior, worse from heat, better from cold open air, thirstless, thick yellow/yellow-greenish discharge, worse after sunset
Sul	Purple appearance, itching is worse from scratching, nostrils are red, very thirsty, cough, diarrhea, worse	This remedy has an affinity for the heart and skin. Worse standing still/heat of bed/water/11am, better

	from early morning	perspiring/motion/dry weather, burning sensations all over body, eczema, craves sweets and open air, children look like they have a potbelly, children hate to take baths

MUMPS

REMEDIES:

Aconite, Belladonna, Jaborandi, Lycopodium, Mercurius Sol., Phytolacca, Pulsatilla, Rhus Tox.

Remedy	Symptom Differentiation	Keynote Differentiation
Acon	Beginning stages of mumps, sudden onset, high fever, restlessness, anxiety, thirsty	This remedy has an affinity for the circulatory and nervous system. Worse extreme or sudden cold/extreme heat/night, better with perspiration, rapid pulse, sudden high fever, red skin, intense thirst for large quantities of cold water, restlessness, anxiety, fear of death, croup cough
Bell	Flushed face, headache is throbbing, glands are swollen and hot, drowsy, insomnia	Symptoms usually have sudden and violent onset, local congestion of blood (example face is red), the congested area is usually hot, children usually convulse when they have a fever
Jab	Glands are swollen and painful, pain spreads to breasts and ovaries, face is red, profuse saliva and sweat	Saliva and perspiration is profuse
Lyc	Swelling moves from right to left	This remedy has an affinity for liver and digestion, kidneys and genitals, mucus and skin, and nervous system. Worse between 4-8pm, worse with heat, better with cool air,

		craving for sweets and oysters, ravenous appetite, flatulence, bloating after meals, doesn't like tight clothes on waist, abdomen is distended, red face after eating, migraine from poor digestion, bedwetting, nose stuffy with crusty mucus especially at night, sleep with mouth open, runny nose during day, anorexia in children
Merc Sol	Glands swollen on right side, saliva and sweat smell foul, worse from blowing nose	This remedy has an affinity for the digestive and renal systems with specific action on throat. Foul-smelling breath, gums are white/yellow color and ulcers in gums, tooth abscess, sores in mouth, intense thirst, thick tongue, salivate heavily, parotiditis, heavy perspiration especially at night and offensive in odor, ulcers, worse at night, known as "the human thermometer," shivering and goose-bumps
Phyt	Glands are hard like stones, worse from cold/wet weather/right side, pain goes to ear, clamps teeth shut, sticking tongue out hurts	This remedy has an affinity for the mucus, breasts and bones. Worse with cold/wet/motion, better with dry weather and resting. Stiffness and bruising all over body, sciatica
Puls	Mumps at late age (especially at puberty), breasts or testicles swollen, thirstless, worse from warm room	This remedy has an affinity for the venous system and mucus. Changeable behavior, worse from heat, better from cold open air, thirstless, thick yellow/yellow-greenish discharge, worse after sunset
Rhus Tox	Glands are swollen, worse on left side and from cold, cold sores	This remedy has an affinity for the skin, mucus and the nervous system. Better with slow motion and changing of position, shivers when slights

		part of body is uncovered, perspiration all over body except the face, sprains and dislocations, worse 4-5am and 7pm, intense thirst for cold water or milk

NAVAL PROBLEMS/UMBILICAL HERNIA

REMEDIES:

Calcarea Carb., Lachesis, Nux Vomica, Opium, Plumbum,

Remedy	Symptom Differentiation	Keynote Differentiation
Calc Carb	Painful to the touch	Any Calcarea remedy has an affinity for bones, lymph nodes, circulation and polyps. They sweat profusely on head, babies teethe late, walk slow and are lazy, large appetite, remember the four F's: fat, fair skin, fainting, and fearful. If Ruta and Rhus Tox have stopped working, this remedy can be thought of. For chronic indications of pulsatilla
Lach	Painful to touch, cannot wear clothing around waist area	This remedy has an affinity for the nervous system and blood. Bruising, hemorrhaging, blotchy face, talkative, suspicious, jealous, spiteful, depression, worse from discharges that are delayed or insufficient/being touched/sun/heat/sleeping/tight clothes/left side, better from discharge that finally comes out, insomnia (especially before midnight), dreams of ghosts, dead people, coffins, difficulty swallowing, sinusitis, apnea, hot flushes in head, ulcers, bed sores
Nux Vom	Very sensitive to pressure, feels bruised and sore, strangulated hernia	This remedy as an affinity for the nervous and digestive system. Irritable, cold, hypersensitive,

		angry, worse after eating, better with sleep, tongue is yellow/white color, craves spicy and sour food, constipation, sneezing upon waking
Op	Incarcerated hernia	This remedy has an affinity for the brain. Coma-like sleep, dark red or purple face, hot perspiration, slow breathing, slow pulse, hypersensitivity of ears, worse from heat/fear/strong emotion, better from cold, absence of pain
Plum	Pain causes desire to stretch	This remedy has an affinity for the digestive, circulatory and nervous system. Gums are swollen/blue/black, teeth loose and smell bad, colic with bloating, constipation, worse with moving around, better with strong pressure and bending forward, muscle paralysis, neuralgic pains, trembling

NOSEBLEEDS

REMEDIES:

Ipecac, Phosphorus

Remedy	Symptom Differentiation	Keynote Differentiation
Ipecac	Bright red blood, nausea, faintness, needs to be fanned	This remedy has an affinity for the digestive and respiratory system. Hemorrhaging bright red blood, profuse saliva, not thirsty at all, disgusted by food, persistent and violent nausea, vomit is sticky and does not relieve nausea, stools are fermented like yeast, cough with suffocation, large amount of mucus

Phos	Frequent nosebleeds, dental hemorrheage	This remedy is highly sensitive especially to light, noises, and smells. Fear of thunderstorm, worse from cold/storms/left side, better from sleep, craves salt and cold drinks, midnight "snacker" especially around 3 am, #1 morning sickness remedy

OTITS MEDIA (EAR INFECTION)

REMEDIES:

Aconite, Belladonna, Chamomilla, Ferrum Phos.

Remedy	Symptom Differentiation	Keynote Differentiation
Acon	Ear infection from cold wind or sudden change of temperature, sudden onset, high fever, ear is hot/red/painful/swollen, sensitive to noise and touch, cheeks are red/hot/swollen/flushed, after 24 hours consider different remedy, worse from warmth/warm room/night, better from open air	This remedy has an affinity for the circulatory and nervous system. Worse extreme or sudden cold/extreme heat/night, better with perspiration, rapid pulse, sudden high fever, red skin, intense thirst for large quantities of cold water, restlessness, anxiety, fear of death, croup cough
Bell	Sudden onset, early stages of ear infection, skin is hot/red/flushed face, eyes are glaring, senses are hypersensitive, thirstless, ear/eardrum/ear canal is red, ear pain extends to throat, high fever	Symptoms usually have sudden and violent onset, local congestion of blood (example face is red), the congested area is usually hot, children usually convulse when they have a fever
Cham	Stabbing pain in ear, sudden onset, ear infection during teething, worse from heat/opn air/cold/wind/touch/eating/warmth	This remedy has an affinity for the digestive system. Hypersensitive to pain, pain feels

	of bed/lying down/night, better from being rocked/carried/warm/wet weather/cold compresses	intolerable, numbness, irritable, angry, moody, hateful, exhausted from teething, insomnia, one cheek is red and hot while other is pale and cold, worse from anger/9pm and 12am/heat(toothache), better from being carried or riding in car
Ferr Phos	Sudden onset, ear drum is red and bulging	Tired, anemic, pale. Bleeds easily, low temperature, rapid pulse, face is red and pale alternatingly, hemorrhages easily, better with slow motion, craves sour things

POISON IVY

REMEDIES:

Anacardium, Croton Tig, Graphites, Ledum, Rhus Tox., Sepia, Sulphur

Reme dy	Symptom Differentiation	Keynote Differentiation
Anac	Excessive redness/itching/burning, worse from scratching, better from rubbing/warm compresses/eating, irritable, cursing, antidote to poison ivy	This remedy has an affinity for the nervous system. Senses are weak, does not want to work, cursing, feels like a plug is in certain body parts, feels "plugged up", empty feeling in stomach, worse with hot compresses, better from eating/lying on side/rubbing
Crot Tig	Skin feels tight/red/blisters/oozing/yellow scabs, goes from itching-scratching-burning, better after sleep, antidote to poison ivy	This remedy has an affinity for the skin and rectum. Eyes feel drawn back, stools forcibly shoot out, chest pain drawing to the back, worse from food/drink/summer/touch/night/morning/washing

Graph	Skin erupts thick/glutinous/sticky/honey-colored, skin is itching/burning/stitching, worse from wearing clothing/heat/water/night	This remedy has similar properties to the Calcarea family of remedies. Anemia with redness of face, obesity tendency, cries from music, head pain is burning on top of head, eyelids have eczema/red/swollen, moisture and rash behind ears, hissing noises in ear, stomach pain is constrictive/burning/causes hunger, loosens clothing, rashes ooze, unhealthy skin, worse from warmth and night, better from dark and being wrapped up
Led	Skin is itching, better from cold water	This remedy has an affinity for the joints and the skin. Rheumatism, poison-ivy-like rash, tetanus, twitching, better from cold, worse at night and from heat of bed
Rhus Tox	Skin is itching/burning/stinging/pus, worse from scratching/night/warmth of bed, better from hot water	This remedy has an affinity for the skin, mucus and the nervous system. Better with slow motion and changing of position, shivers when slights part of body is uncovered, perspiration all over body except the face, sprains and dislocations, worse 4-5am and 7pm, intense thirst for cold water or milk
Sep	Skin color is yellow, itching gives no relief	This remedy has an affinity for the circulatory and nervous system. Hormonal imbalance. Sitting or kneeling for long periods causes fainting, worse before storm, better with exercise, feels like abdomen is heavy, flushes of heat in face, craves vinegar, and sour foods, worse 11 am
Sul	Skin burns and itches, worse from warm bath, better from scratching (especially until it bleeds)	This remedy has an affinity for the heart and skin. Worse standing still/heat of bed/water/11am, better perspiring/motion/dry weather, burning sensations all over body, eczema, craves sweets and open air, children look like they have a potbelly, children hate to take baths

RESTLESSNESS/FUSSY

REMEDIES:

Argentrum Nitricum, Arsenicum Album, Chamomilla, Coffea Nux Vomica, Rhus Tox.

Reme dy	Symptom Differentiation	Keynote Differentiation
Arg Nit	Agitated, impulsive, anxious, worse from heat	This remedy has an affinity for the nervous system and the mucus. Nervousness, "what-if," feels as if a thorn is stuck certain part of body, feels like head is expanding, feels squeezing sensation, worse from heat/eating candy/intellectual work/right side, better from fresh air and pressure, vertigo, anticipation anxiety (especially for tests), stomach ulcers
Ars	High strung, nervous, easily startled, anxious, pacing, fussy, scared of being alone and dark	This remedy has an affinity for mucus, kidneys liver, adrenal glands and the nervous system. This remedy can be summed up in three words: weak, restless and cold (temperature-wise). Burning pains, worse 1-3am and

		from the cold, thirsty for small amounts of cold water, fear of death, food-poisoning
Cham	Temper tantrums, refuses things asked for, nothing satisfies only being carried or rocked	This remedy has an affinity for the digestive system. Hypersensitive to pain, pain feels intolerable, numbness, irritable, angry, moody, hateful, exhausted from teething, insomnia, one cheek is red and hot while other is pale and cold, worse from anger/9pm and 12am/heat(toothache), better from being carried or riding in car
Coff	Breast-feeding mother drinks coffee	This remedy has an affinity for hyperactivity especially of the mind. Intolerance to pain, toothache better from cold water
Nux Vom	Hyperactivity, over-excitable, temper tantrums, sensitive to touch/pain/noise/odors/music/food/medication, angry when woken up	This remedy as an affinity for the nervous and digestive system. Irritable, cold, hypersensitive, angry, worse after eating, better with sleep, tongue is

		yellow/white color, craves spicy and sour food, constipation, sneezing upon waking
Rhus Tox	Constantly moving, worse at night, tosses and turns	This remedy has an affinity for the skin, mucus and the nervous system. Better with slow motion and changing of position, shivers when slights part of body is uncovered, perspiration all over body except the face, sprains and dislocations, worse 4-5am and 7pm, intense thirst for cold water or milk

RINGWORM

REMEDIES:

Calcarea Carb., Thuja

Remedy	Symptom Differentiation	Keynote Differentiation
Calc Carb	#1 Remedy for Ringworm	Any Calcarea remedy has an affinity for bones, lymph nodes, circulation and polyps. They sweat profusely on head, babies teethe late, walk slow and are lazy, large appetite, remember the four F's: fat, fair skin, fainting, and fearful. If Ruta and Rhus Tox have stopped working, this remedy can be thought of. For chronic

		indications of pulsatilla
Thuja	Ringworm with discoloration of skin in patches	This remedy has an affinity for the skin, mucus, and any type of growths appearing inside of body or outside on the skin: warts, moles, acne, seborrhea, cradle cap, hair loss, scalp has white scaly dandruff Worse cold/humid weather/3 am or 3 pm, better with heat, discharges have a moldy smell

R.S.V.

REMEDIES:

Antimonium Tart., Belladonna, Cuprum, Hyoscyamus, Ipecacuanha, Lobelia, Lycopodium, Pulsatilla, Stramonium

Remedy	Symptom Differentiation	Keynote Differentiation
Ant Tart	Nostrils flaring (because of congestion and not enough air), mucus is ratting in chest, gas and bloating	This remedy has an affinity for the respiratory system and the skin. This remedy can be summed up with three words: exhaustion, paleness, and sleepiness. Spitting behavior, grasps for other people
Bell	RSV from cool exposure, sudden onset, spasms, worse from 3am-3pm, better from rest and in the dark, worse from cold air	Symptoms usually have sudden and violent onset, local congestion of blood (example face is red), the congested area is usually hot, children usually convulse when they have a fever
Cup	Bronchial spasms, cramps, better from warmth/rest/cold drinks, worse at night	This remedy has an affinity for the muscular system. Spasmodic pain begins and ends suddenly, convulsions, blue face, violent cramping, whooping cough, better drinking a sip of cold water, violent diarrhea with cramping pains
Hyos	Irritability, bronchial	This remedy has an affinity for

	spasms, worse from cold/lying down/stimulation, better from warmth/sitting/moving around	the nervous system. Laughs at everything, uncovers body, jealous, foolish, attempting to run away, muttering speech, quarrelsome, sobs and cries without waking up, worse at night/after eating/lying down
Ipecac	Coughing until vomiting, tongue looks clean	This remedy has an affinity for the digestive and respiratory system. Hemorrhaging bright red blood, profuse saliva, not thirsty at all, disgusted by food, persistent and violent nausea, vomit is sticky and does not relieve nausea, stools are fermented like yeast, cough with suffocation, large amount of mucus
Lob	Bronchial spasms, weakness, cold sweat, pale face, asthma and rsv comes on slowly, worse from cold compresses, better from warmth	Prickling sensation all over body, weakness in pit of stomach, lump feeling in sternum
Lyc	Nose is flaring, worse from 4-8pm	This remedy has an affinity for liver and digestion, kidneys and genitals, mucus and skin, and nervous system. Worse between 4-8pm, worse with heat, better with cool air, craving for sweets and oysters, ravenous appetite, flatulence, bloating after meals, doesn't like tight clothes on waist, abdomen is distended, red face after eating, migraine from poor digestion, bedwetting, nose stuffy with crusty mucus especially at night, sleep with mouth open, runny nose during day, anorexia in children
Puls	Mucus is thick/creamy/changeable,	This remedy has an affinity for the venous system and mucus.

	better from open air	Changeable behavior, worse from heat, better from cold open air, thirstless, thick yellow/yellow-greenish discharge, worse after sunset
Stram	Bronchial spasms, irritable, head feels hot, feet are ice cold, worse from the dark, better from light	This remedy has an affinity for the brain and the nervous system. Worse in dark/shinny and bright objects/being alone, better from soft light and being around people, severe and violent convulsions, incoherent talkativeness, hallucinations, nightmares, swollen tongue, doesn't like the sight of liquids, spasmodic and suffocative cough, bright red rash

ROSEOLA

REMEDIES:

Aconite, Bryonia, Pulsatilla

Remedy	Symptom Differentiation	Keynote Differentiation
Acon		This remedy has an affinity for the circulatory and nervous system. Worse extreme or sudden cold/extreme heat/night, better with perspiration, rapid pulse, sudden high fever, red skin, intense thirst for large quantities of cold water, restlessness, anxiety, fear of death, croup cough
Bry		Very thirsty especially if during a fever, sinuses are very dry (hint to remember: if dry think "bry"), pressure headaches that usually travel from forehead to occiput, or can start from left eye and move to the back of the

		head
Puls		This remedy has an affinity for the venous system and mucus. Changeable behavior, worse from heat, better from cold open air, thirstless, thick yellow/yellow-greenish discharge, worse after sunset

SCREAMING

REMEDIES:

Aconite, Antimonium Tart., Belladonna, Borax, Calcarea Phos., Chamomilla, China, Cina, Coffea, Kali Phos., Kreosotum, Lycopodium, Nux Vomica, Rheum

Remedy	Symptom Differentiation	Keynote Differentiation
Acon	Screaming with pain	This remedy has an affinity for the circulatory and nervous system. Worse extreme or sudden cold/extreme heat/night, better with perspiration, rapid pulse, sudden high fever, red skin, intense thirst for large quantities of cold water, restlessness, anxiety, fear of death, croup cough
Ant Tart	Screaming if touched	This remedy has an affinity for the respiratory system and the skin. This remedy can be summed up with three words: exhaustion, paleness, and sleepiness. Spitting behavior, grasps for other people
Bell	Screaming with pain	Symptoms usually have sudden and violent onset, local congestion of blood (example face is red), the congested area is usually hot, children usually convulse when they have a fever
Bor	Screaming during sleep	This remedy has an affinity for

		the nervous system, skin and mucus of the mouth. Thrush, aphthae of mouth, refuse to eat because painful patches inside cheeks, skin looks unhealthy, worse leaning forward/downward/falling motion
Calc Phos	Screaming in sleep	This remedy has an affinity for the bones, blood, lymph nodes and works on the nutrition of the body. Teeth are long, narrow and yellow, bones are long and straight, tired and nervous, rickets, weight loss, repetitive sore throat/bronchitis/colds
Cham	Screaming with pain and on waking	This remedy has an affinity for the digestive system. Hypersensitive to pain, pain feels intolerable, numbness, irritable, angry, moody, hateful, exhausted from teething, insomnia, one cheek is red and hot while other is pale and cold, worse from anger/9pm and 12am/heat(toothache), better from being carried or riding in car
China	Screaming on waking	This remedy is known for ringing and buzzing in ears, hypersensitivity of senses, hypotension, bitter taste in mouth, gas, worse from drafts/slight pressure/every other day/beer/milk/fruit, better from heat and strong pressure, no appetite, loss of vital fluids, pulsating headaches, hemorrhages
Cina	Screaming on waking	Convulsions beginning on one side of the face, attack stops and begins at the same time,

		breathing slows down, urine incontinence, do not like to be touched or looked at, large circles under the eyes, sickly appearance, yawn frequently, grinding of teeth, restless sleep, frequent rubbing of nose and scratching of nostrils, constant hunger that is not easily satiable, pain in belly-button better by lying on abdomen, worse during new moon and full moon, better lying on stomach/abdomen, presence of round worms, teething
Coff	Screaming with pain	This remedy has an affinity for hyperactivity especially of the mind. Intolerance to pain, toothache better from cold water
Kali Phos	Screaming on waking	This remedy has an affinity for the nervous and muscular system as well as the blood. Weak, tired, and hypersensitive, worse over-nursing and over-stimulation of mind, discharges are golden, orange or bloody, irritable, moody, headaches in children, nightmares cause insomnia, vaginitis with brown discharge
Kreos	Screaming in newborn	This remedy has an affinity for mucus and tends to hemorrhage.
Lyc	Screaming in newborn/on waking/during sleep	This remedy has an affinity for liver and digestion, kidneys and genitals, mucus and skin, and nervous system. Worse between 4-8pm, worse with heat, better with cool air, craving for sweets and oysters, ravenous appetite, flatulence, bloating after meals, doesn't like

		tight clothes on waist, abdomen is distended, red face after eating, migraine from poor digestion, bedwetting, nose stuffy with crusty mucus especially at night, sleep with mouth open, runny nose during day, anorexia in children
Nux Vom	Irritability, angry, grumpy	This remedy as an affinity for the nervous and digestive system. Irritable, cold, hypersensitive, angry, worse after eating, better with sleep, tongue is yellow/white color, craves spicy and sour food, constipation, sneezing upon waking
Rheum		This remedy has an affinity for the liver and intestines. Great teething remedy- restless/temperamental/scalp perspiration, cries when passing stool, sour smell from whole body

SKIN PROBLEMS/ACNE

REMEDIES:

Antimonium Crudum, Belladonna, Berberis, Ledum, Nux Vomica, Sulphur, Thuja

Remedy	Symptom Differentiation	Keynote Differentiation
Ant Crud	pimples, vesicles, scabs are thick/hard/honey-colored, looks like measles, warts, skin is dry/scaly/burning/itching, worse at night and cold baths	This remedy has an affinity for the digestive tract, especially the stomach, and the skin. Tongue has thick white coating, thrush, burping, watery diarrhea,

		impetigo, warts, thick and hard nails, worse cold bath/radiating heat/over-eating
Bell	Skin is dry/hot/swollen/sensitive/scarlet red/smooth, boils, acne, rosacea	Symptoms usually have sudden and violent onset, local congestion of blood (example face is red), the congested area is usually hot, children usually convulse when they have a fever
Berb	Skin is itching and burning, small pimples over whole body, flat warts, worse from scratching, better from cold compresses	Changeable symptoms: thirsty then thirstless, hungry then no appetite, gout, feels like a cap is over head, nausea before breakfast, thick and red urine, neuralgia under finger nails, worse from motion/standing /scratching
Led	Acne on forehead, facial eczema, worse from scratching and warmth of bed	This remedy has an affinity for the joints and the skin. Rheumatism, poison-ivy-like rash, tetanus, twitching, better from cold, worse at night and from heat of bed
Nux Vom	Skin is burning hot (especially face), acne, red and blotching skin	This remedy as an affinity for the nervous and digestive system. Irritable, cold, hypersensitive,

			angry, worse after eating, better with sleep, tongue is yellow/white color, craves spicy and sour food, constipation, sneezing upon waking
Sul		Skin is dry/scaly/unhealthy/freckles/itching/burning, worse from scratching/washing/warmth, hang nails	This remedy has an affinity for the heart and skin. Worse standing still/heat of bed/water/11am, better perspiring/motion/ dry weather, burning sensations all over body, eczema, craves sweets and open air, children look like they have a potbelly, children hate to take baths
Thuja		Skin is dry with brown spots, eruptions come out on covered areas, warts, polyps, nevi, freckles, blotches	This remedy has an affinity for the skin, mucus, and any type of growths appearing inside of body or outside on the skin: warts, moles, acne, seborrhea, cradle cap, hair loss, scalp has white scaly dandruff Worse cold/humid weather/3 am or 3 pm, better with heat, discharges have a moldy smell

SKIN PROBLEMS/DRY SKIN

REMEDIES:

Aconite, Alumina, Arsenicum Album, Belladonna, Graphites, Plumbum

Remedy	Symptom Differentiation	Keynote Differentiation
Acon	Skin is red/hot/swollen/dry/burning, feeling of ants, numbness	This remedy has an affinity for the circulatory and nervous system. Worse extreme or sudden cold/extreme heat/night, better with perspiration, rapid pulse, sudden high fever, red skin, intense thirst for large quantities of cold water, restlessness, anxiety, fear of death, croup cough
Alu	Skin is chapped and dry, brittle nails, scratches until bleeds, brittle skin on fingers, intolerable itching when getting into warm bed	This remedy has an affinity for the skin and mucus. Weakness, dryness, wrinkled, afraid of sharp instruments and blood, extreme constipation, worse in morning and after eating potatoes, better open air and wearing warm clothes
Ars	Skin is itching/burning/swollen/dry/rough/scaly, worse from cold and scratching	This remedy has an affinity for mucus, kidneys liver, adrenal glands and the nervous system. This remedy can be summed up in three words: weak, restless and cold

		(temperature-wise). Burning pains, worse 1-3am and from the cold, thirsty for small amounts of cold water, fear of death, food-poisoning
Bell	Skin is dry/hot swollen, boils	Symptoms usually have sudden and violent onset, local congestion of blood (example face is red), the congested area is usually hot, children usually convulse when they have a fever
Grap h	Skin is rough/hard/dry/keloids/pimples/acne/e czema/raw (especially behind the ears)/cracked/unhealthy, discharge is yellow/thick/oozing	This remedy has similar properties to the Calcarea family of remedies. Anemia with redness of face, obesity tendency, cries from music, head pain is burning on top of head, eyelids have eczema/red/swollen, moisture and rash behind ears, hissing noises in ear, stomach pain is constrictive/burning/ causes hunger, loosens clothing, rashes ooze, unhealthy skin, worse from warmth and night, better from dark and being wrapped up
Plum	Skin is yellow with dark-brown liver spots	This remedy has an affinity for the digestive, circulatory

		and nervous system. Gums are swollen/blue/black, teeth loose and smell bad, colic with bloating, constipation, worse with moving around, better with strong pressure and bending forward, muscle paralysis, neuralgic pains, trembling

SKIN PROBLEMS/ECZEMA

REMEDIES:

Antimonium Crudum, Arsenicum Album, Calcarea Carb., Croton Tig., Graphites, Mezereum, Silica, Sulphur

Remedy	Symptom Differentiation	Keynote Differentiation
Ant Crud	Eczema from stomach issues, pimples, vesicles, scabs are thick/hard/honey-colored, looks like measles, warts, skin is dry/scaly/burning/itching, worse at night and cold baths	This remedy has an affinity for the digestive tract, especially the stomach, and the skin. Tongue has thick white coating, thrush, burping, watery diarrhea, impetigo, warts, thick and hard nails, worse cold bath/radiating heat/over-eating
Ars	Skin is itching/burning/swollen/dry/rough/scaly, worse from cold and scratching	This remedy has an affinity for mucus, kidneys liver, adrenal glands and the nervous system. This remedy can be summed up in three words: weak, restless and cold (temperature-wise). Burning pains, worse 1-3am and from the cold, thirsty for small amounts of cold water, fear of death, food-poisoning
Calc Carb	Skin is unhealthy, doesn't heal well, warts,	Any Calcarea remedy has an affinity for bones, lymph nodes, circulation

40

	boils, better in cold air	and polyps. They sweat profusely on head, babies teethe late, walk slow and are lazy, large appetite, remember the four F's: fat, fair skin, fainting, and fearful. If Ruta and Rhus Tox have stopped working, this remedy can be thought of. For chronic indications of pulsatilla
Crot Tig	Skin feels tight/red/blisters/oozing/yellow scabs, goes from itching-scratching-burning, better after sleep, antidote to poison ivy	This remedy has an affinity for the skin and rectum. Eyes feel drawn back, stools forcibly shoot out, chest pain drawing to the back, worse from food/drink/summer/touch/night/morning/washing
Graph	Skin is rough/hard/dry/keloids/pimples/acne/eczema/raw (especially behind the ears)/cracked/unhealthy, discharge is yellow/thick/oozing	This remedy has similar properties to the Calcarea family of remedies. Anemia with redness of face, obesity tendency, cries from music, head pain is burning on top of head, eyelids have eczema/red/swollen, moisture and rash behind ears, hissing noises in ear, stomach pain is constrictive/burning/causes hunger, loosens clothing, rashes ooze, unhealthy skin, worse from warmth and night, better from dark and being wrapped up
Mez	Eczema with intolerable itching, skin is itching/burning/shining/red/thick scabs/swollen, worse from damp weather/touch/night	This remedy has an affinity for the bones and the skin. Joints feel bruised and stiff, skin problems after vaccines, very sensitive to cold air, crusts on head look like leather, facial neuralgia, worse from cold air/night/until midnight/warm food/touch/motion, better from open air
Sil	Skin is prone to abscesses/boils/ulcers/looks delicate/pale/waxy/cracks (especially end of	This remedy has an affinity for the nervous system and is very malnourished. They are weak and demineralized. Worse cold and humid weather, better with heat,

	fingers)/blotches/keloids, itchy in daytime and evening	slinters (will push them out), fontanels stay open, perspire on head, abscess remedy, white spots on nails, weak nails/hair
Sul	Skin is dry/scaly/unhealthy/freckles/itching/burning, worse from scratching/washing/warmth, hang nails	This remedy has an affinity for the heart and skin. Worse standing still/heat of bed/water/11am, better perspiring/motion/dry weather, burning sensations all over body, eczema, craves sweets and open air, children look like they have a potbelly, children hate to take baths

SORE THROAT

REMEDIES:

Aconite, Apis, Arsenicum Album, Belladonna, Ferrum Phos., Hepar Sulph., Ignatia, Lachesis, Lycopodium, Mercurius Sol., Mercurius Iodatus Rub., Mercuruius Iodatus Flavus, Phytolacca, Rhus Tox., Sulphur, Wyethia

Remedy	Symptom Differentiation	Keynote Differentiation
Acon	Beginning stage of sore throat, sudden symptoms, sore throat from cold air, throat is burning/red/dry/swollen	This remedy has an affinity for the circulatory and nervous system. Worse extreme or sudden cold/extreme heat/night, better with perspiration, rapid pulse, sudden high fever, red skin, intense thirst for large quantities of cold water, restlessness, anxiety, fear of death, croup cough
Apis	Throat is shiny/red/inflamed/dry/burning/stinging, worse from warm drinks and warm food, better from cold drinks and ice cubes, hoarseness in the morning, feels like a fishbone is in throat, difficulty swallowing	This remedy is known for swelling, burning pain, and jealousy. Worse from heat, better from cold, hot dry skin, inflammation

42

Ars	Throat is burning, mouth is dry, thirsty for sups of water, worse from cold food and cold drinks, better from warm food and warm drinks. Started with nasal discharge, then moves into throat.	This remedy has an affinity for mucus, kidneys liver, adrenal glands and the nervous system. This remedy can be summed up in three words: weak, restless and cold (temperature-wise). Burning pains, worse 1-3am and from the cold, thirsty for small amounts of cold water, fear of death, food-poisoning
Bell	Throat is scarlet red, burning pain, desire to swallow but hurts, constriction in throat, desires lemonade, ticking in larynx	Symptoms usually have sudden and violent onset, local congestion of blood (example face is red), the congested area is usually hot, children usually convulse when they have a fever
Ferr Phos	Throat is red/burning/swollen, worse on waking up, better with cold, difficulty swallowing, hoarseness, over-use of voice	Tired, anemic, pale. Bleeds easily, low temperature, rapid pulse, face is red and pale alternatingly, hemorrhages easily, better with slow motion, craves sour things
Hep Sul	Feels like stick is in throat, sore throat after cold, difficulty swallowing, pain goes to ear, better with hot drinks	This remedy is hypersensitive especially to touch and cold air, worse dry/cold weather/slightest draft, better with heat, craves sour things especially vinegar
Ign	Sore throat better by swallowing food, worse swallowing saliva, fells like lump is in throat, hoarseness, loss of voice	This remedy is hypersensitive on all organs and senses especially sight and hearing. Very sensitive emotionally especially to sad events, spasms, uncoordinated, sensitive to any sort of excitement or

		pain, nervous behavior, sighing, fainting, moody, outbreaks of anger, cries easily, irritability, weakness, feels like lump in throat, migraines feel like nails in head, worse 11am/sad news/being consoled/strong smells, better from heat and good time with company, nervous breakdown
Lach	Tickle or fishbone feeling in throat, worse swallowing saliva/warm liquids/left side/coughing up mucus	This remedy has an affinity for the nervous system and blood. Bruising, hemorrhaging, blotchy face, talkative, suspicious, jealous, spiteful, depression, worse from discharges that are delayed or insufficient/being touched/sun/heat/sleeping /tight clothes/left side, better from discharge that finally comes out, insomnia (especially before midnight), dreams of ghosts, dead people, coffins, difficulty swallowing, sinusitis, apnea, hot flushes in head, ulcers, bed sores
Lyc	Sore throat starts on right then left, right is more inflamed, worse from cold liquids, better from warm liquids, choking, feels like ball in throat	This remedy has an affinity for liver and digestion, kidneys and genitals, mucus and skin, and nervous system. Worse between 4-8pm, worse with heat, better with cool air, craving for sweets and oysters, ravenous appetite, flatulence, bloating after meals, doesn't like tight

		clothes on waist, abdomen is distended, red face after eating, migraine from poor digestion, bedwetting, nose stuffy with crusty mucus especially at night, sleep with mouth open, runny nose during day, anorexia in children
Merc Sol	Desire to swallow but hurts, choking from swallowing, throat is red/swollen/raw/burning/dry, saliva profuse, breath is foul	This remedy has an affinity for the digestive and renal systems with specific action on throat. Foul-smelling breath, gums are white/yellow color and ulcers in gums, tooth abscess, sores in mouth, intense thirst, thick tongue, salivate heavily, parotiditis, heavy perspiration especially at night and offensive in odor, ulcers, worse at night, known as "the human thermometer," shivering and goose-bumps
MIR	Sore throat on the left, desire to swallow but hurts, choking from swallowing, throat is red/swollen/raw/burning/dry, saliva profuse, breath is foul	This remedy has an affinity for the digestive and renal systems with specific action on throat. Foul-smelling breath, gums are white/yellow color and ulcers in gums, tooth abscess, sores in mouth, intense thirst, thick tongue, salivate heavily, parotiditis, heavy perspiration especially at night and offensive in odor, ulcers, worse at night, known as "the human thermometer," shivering and goose-bumps
MIF	Sore throat on the right, desire to swallow but hurts, choking	This remedy has an affinity for the digestive and renal

	from swallowing, throat is red/swollen/raw/burning/dry, saliva profuse, breath is foul	systems with specific action on throat. Foul-smelling breath, gums are white/yellow color and ulcers in gums, tooth abscess, sores in mouth, intense thirst, thick tongue, salivate heavily, parotiditis, heavy perspiration especially at night and offensive in odor, ulcers, worse at night, known as "the human thermometer," shivering and goose-bumps
Phyt	Throat pain shoots from throat to ears, pain in roof of tongue causes tongue to stick out, throat is raw/rough/swollen/constricted, worse on right side, neck glands are swollen	This remedy has an affinity for the mucus, breasts and bones. Worse with cold/wet/motion, better with dry weather and resting. Stiffness and bruising all over body, sciatica
Rhus Tox	Throat is sore with swollen glands, sticking pain on swallowing, worse on left side	This remedy has an affinity for the skin, mucus and the nervous system. Better with slow motion and changing of position, shivers when slights part of body is uncovered, perspiration all over body except the face, sprains and dislocations, worse 4-5am and 7pm, intense thirst for cold water or milk
Sul	Pressure in throat like a lump/splinter/hair, throat is burning/red/dry	This remedy has an affinity for the heart and skin. Worse standing still/heat of bed/water/11am, better perspiring/motion/dry weather, burning sensations all over body, eczema, craves sweets and open air, children look like they have

		a potbelly, children hate to take baths
Wye	Constantly clearing of throat, dry/swollen/burning, difficulty swallowing, desire to swallow saliva	This remedy has an affinity for the throat. Irritable throat from singers and public speakers, hemorrhoids, hayfever

SPLINTERS

REMEDIES:

Hepar Sulph., Silica

Remedy	Symptom Differentiation	Keynote Differentiation
Hep Sul	Imbedded splinters that cannot be removed with tweezers (give Silica 1ˢᵗ)	This remedy is hypersensitive especially to touch and cold air, worse dry/cold weather/slightest draft, better with heat, craves sour things especially vinegar
Sil	#1 Remedy to expel splinters under skin, wound is inflamed	This remedy has an affinity for the nervous system and is very malnourished. They are weak and demineralized. Worse cold and humid weather, better with heat, slinters (will push them out), fontanels stay open, perspire on head, abscess remedy, white spots on nails, weak nails/hair

SPRAINS

REMEDIES:

Arnica, Bellis Perenis, Bryonia, Calcarea Carb., Ledum, Rhus Tox., Ruta

Remedy	Symptom Differentiation	Keynote Differentiation
Arn	#1 Remedy for any injury. To be given	This remedy has an affinity for the muscles, capillaries and cellular tissues.

	1st, secondary remedy for specific injury, keeps swelling down	Contusions, stiffness, muscular pain, feel that bed is too hard, worse from slightest touch/jolt/movement/damp cold, better from lying with head lower than feet, #1 trauma remedy/accidents/falls/hemorrhaging, given to stop bleeding. If you have children, you will give this remedy to your child several times throughout their childhood. For falls and bleeding, give the highest potency you have.
Bell Per	Severe sprains	This remedy has an affinity for the muscles. Lameness, sprained feeling, good remedy after surgery, gout, worse from cold baths, boils, acne, varicose veins
Bry	Injury worse with motion	Very thirsty especially if during a fever, sinuses are very dry (hint to remember: if dry think "bry"), pressure headaches that usually travel from forehead to occiput, or can start from left eye and move to the back of the head
Calc Carb	Injury to hand, wrist, ankle, worse lifting	Any Calcarea remedy has an affinity for bones, lymph nodes, circulation and polyps. They sweat profusely on head, babies teethe late, walk slow and are lazy, large appetite, remember the four F's: fat, fair skin, fainting, and fearful. If Ruta and Rhus Tox have stopped working, this remedy can be thought of. For chronic indications of pulsatilla
Led	Sprain easily especially ankles	This remedy has an affinity for the joints and the skin. Rheumatism, poison-ivy-like rash, tetanus, twitching, better from cold, worse at night and from heat of bed
Rhus Tox	Heals sprain, stiff, painful, loosens up with continuous motion, worse from over-exertion	This remedy has an affinity for the skin, mucus and the nervous system. Better with slow motion and changing of position, shivers when slights part of body is uncovered, perspiration all

48

		over body except the face, sprains and dislocations, worse 4-5am and 7pm, intense thirst for cold water or milk
Ruta	Tearing of tendon, feels hot	Dequervian syndrome, bone injuries, fractures with slow repair of broken bones, affinity for tendons, joints, wrists, ankles, cartilage, periosteum, and skin

TANTRUMS

REMEDIES:

Belladonna, Calcarea Carb., Chamomilla, Lycopodium, Nitricum Acidum, Pulsatilla, Stramonium, Tuberculinum

Remedy	Symptom Differentiation	Keynote Differentiation
Bell	Angry, irritable, flushed, screaming, bites hands, crying	Symptoms usually have sudden and violent onset, local congestion of blood (example face is red), the congested area is usually hot, children usually convulse when they have a fever
Calc Carb	Clings while screaming, holds onto mothers leg	Any Calcarea remedy has an affinity for bones, lymph nodes, circulation and polyps. They sweat profusely on head, babies teethe late, walk slow and are lazy, large appetite, remember the four F's: fat, fair skin, fainting, and fearful. If Ruta and Rhus Tox have stopped working, this remedy can be thought of. For chronic indications of pulsatilla
Cham	Angry, irritable, screaming, hitting, don't know what they want, worse at night, better being carried and rocked	This remedy has an affinity for the digestive system. Hypersensitive to pain, pain feels intolerable, numbness, irritable, angry, moody, hateful, exhausted from teething, insomnia, one cheek is red and hot while other is pale and cold,

		worse from anger/9pm and 12am/heat(toothache), better from being carried or riding in car
Lyc	Dictatorial behavior	This remedy has an affinity for liver and digestion, kidneys and genitals, mucus and skin, and nervous system. Worse between 4-8pm, worse with heat, better with cool air, craving for sweets and oysters, ravenous appetite, flatulence, bloating after meals, doesn't like tight clothes on waist, abdomen is distended, red face after eating, migraine from poor digestion, bedwetting, nose stuffy with crusty mucus especially at night, sleep with mouth open, runny nose during day, anorexia in children
Nit Ac	"Pissed, pest, pessimistic"	This remedy has an affinity for the body's mucus. Worse from cold/noise/night, better from heat and riding in the car, prickling pains, craves fatty foods, lips are cracked in corners, anal fissures, plantar warts
Puls	Runs away and then comes back	This remedy has an affinity for the venous system and mucus. Changeable behavior, worse from heat, better from cold open air, thirstless, thick yellow/yellow-greenish discharge, worse after sunset
Stram	Violent behavior	This remedy has an affinity for the brain and the nervous system. Worse in dark/shinny and bright objects/being alone, better from soft light and being around people, severe and violent convulsions, incoherent

		talkativeness, hallucinations, nightmares, swollen tongue, doesn't like the sight of liquids, spasmodic and suffocative cough, bright red rash
Tub	Desire to run away, irritable, angry, crying, fussy, contrary, destructive, bangs head on floor and wall	Nervous hypersensitivity, rapid weight loss, extreme sensitivity to cold, slow physical development, very dissatisfied, worse from least exercise/standing/change in weather/stuffy room, better from outside/fresh air/rest/continuous movement, cough at night, craving for cold milk even if they are intolerant of, uncontrollable diarrhea at 5am

TEETH PROBLEMS/TEETHING

REMEDIES:

Aconite, Belladonna, Borax, Calcarea Carb., Calcarea Phos., Chamomilla, Coffea, Kreosotum, Magnesia Mur., Magnesia Phos., Phytolacca, Plantago, Pulsatilla, Rheum, Silica

Remedy	Symptom Differentiation	Keynote Differentiation
Acon	Painful teething, cheeks hot and red, fever, restless sleep	This remedy has an affinity for the circulatory and nervous system. Worse extreme or sudden cold/extreme heat/night, better with perspiration, rapid pulse, sudden high fever, red skin, intense thirst for large quantities of cold water, restlessness, anxiety, fear of death, croup cough
Bell	Lips and gums are red and twitching, very painful, kicking, screaming, biting, restlessness	Symptoms usually have sudden and violent onset, local congestion of blood (example face is red), the

		congested area is usually hot, children usually convulse when they have a fever
Bor	Painful teething	This remedy has an affinity for the nervous system, skin and mucus of the mouth. Thrush, aphthae of mouth, refuse to eat because painful patches inside cheeks, skin looks unhealthy, worse leaning forward/downward/falling motion
Calc Carb	Late teething >12 months, head perspires, grinds teeth at night, better from fingers in mouth, diarrhea	Any Calcarea remedy has an affinity for bones, lymph nodes, circulation and polyps. They sweat profusely on head, babies teethe late, walk slow and are lazy, large appetite, remember the four F's: fat, fair skin, fainting, and fearful. If Ruta and Rhus Tox have stopped working, this remedy can be thought of. For chronic indications of pulsatilla
Calc Phos	Late teething >12 months, late milestones, diarrhea, flatulence, green stools	This remedy has an affinity for the bones, blood, lymph nodes and works on the nutrition of the body. Teeth are long, narrow and yellow, bones are long and straight, tired and nervous, rickets, weight loss, repetitive sore throat/bronchitis/colds
Cham	Irritable and impatient, worse from touch, better from fingers in mouth/cold compresses/ice/rocked/carried, green stools smells like rotten eggs, one side of cheek or gum is red	This remedy has an affinity for the digestive system. Hypersensitive to pain, pain feels intolerable, numbness, irritable, angry, moody, hateful, exhausted from teething, insomnia, one cheek is red and hot while other is

		pale and cold, worse from anger/9pm and 12am/heat(toothache), better from being carried or riding in car
Coff	Hyperactive, insomnia	This remedy has an affinity for hyperactivity especially of the mind. Intolerance to pain, toothache better from cold water
Kreos	Severe pain, decay as soon as teeth appear, restless sleep	This remedy has an affinity for mucus and tends to hemorrhage.
Mag Mur	Teething with colic, green stool	This remedy has an affinity for the digestive and uterine system. Worse from salt (eating and being by sea) and drinking milk, better by pressure, tongue has teeth marks, constipation with hard stools like that of sheep droppings, migraines better with wrapping heat with warm compress
Mag Phos	Spasms, better from warm or hot drinks	This remedy has an affinity for the muscular system. It is a spasmodic remedy. Sudden/intolerable/cramping pains, worse from cold and right side, better from heat and leaning forward
Phyt	Crying, biting gums hard	This remedy has an affinity for the mucus, breasts and bones. Worse with cold/wet/motion, better with dry weather and resting. Stiffness and bruising all over body, sciatica
Plant	Ear pain with teething	This remedy has an affinity in treating earache, toothache, and bed-wetting. Sharp pain in eyes, pain between teeth and ears, eyeballs very tender

		to touch, tooth decay, inflammation of middle ear, insomnia
Puls	Better from cold drinks and open air, worse from warm/warmth of bed/hot drinks	This remedy has an affinity for the venous system and mucus. Changeable behavior, worse from heat, better from cold open air, thirstless, thick yellow/yellow-greenish discharge, worse after sunset
Rheum	Diarrhea from teething	This remedy has an affinity for the liver and intestines. Great teething remedy-restless/temperamental/scalp perspiration, cries when passing stool, sour smell from whole body
Sil	Diarrhea from teething, toothache	This remedy has an affinity for the nervous system and is very malnourished. They are weak and demineralized. Worse cold and humid weather, better with heat, slinters (will push them out), fontanels stay open, perspire on head, abscess remedy, white spots on nails, weak nails/hair

TOOTH DECAY

REMEDIES:

Calcarea Fluor., Calcarea Phos., Kreosotum

Remedy	Symptom Differentiation	Keynote Differentiation
Calc Fluor	Unnatural looseness of teeth, with or without pain, loose in sockets, toothache if food touches tooth	Any Calcarea remedy has an affinity for bones, lymph nodes, circulation and polyps. Teeth are irregularly arranged and small in size, and the enamel is poor quality. #1 remedy for bone spurs. Multiple sprains,

		Discharges are usually green or yellow. This remedy is for chronic indications of ruta and rhus tox
Calc Phos	Rapid tooth decay	This remedy has an affinity for the bones, blood, lymph nodes and works on the nutrition of the body. Teeth are long, narrow and yellow, bones are long and straight, tired and nervous, rickets, weight loss, repetitive sore throat/bronchitis/colds
Kreos	Very rapid tooth decay, gums are spongy and bleeding, teeth are dark/crumbling/foul odor/bitter taste	This remedy has an affinity for mucus and tends to hemorrhage.

THRUSH

REMEDIES:

Borax, Hydrastis, Kali Mur., Nat Mur., Mercurius Sol., Sulphuric Acid., Thuja

Remedy	Symptom Differentiation	Keynote Differentiation
Bor	Inside mouth are canker sores/white/hot/dry/bleeds easily/patches, refuses to nurse, worse from touch, excess saliva	This remedy has an affinity for the nervous system, skin and mucus of the mouth. Thrush, aphthae of mouth, refuse to eat because painful patches inside cheeks, skin looks unhealthy, worse leaning forward/downward/falling motion
Hydr	Yellow-coated tongue, yellow mucus	This remedy has an affinity for the mucus membranes. Any discharge is yellow/thick/ropy, muscles are weak, poor digestion, constipation, pain in lower back, emaciated, goiter (especially during puberty),

		smallpox, sinusitis, tongue shows teeth imprint, cannot eat bread or vegetables
Kali Mur	In breastfed babies, white-coated tongue	This remedy has an affinity for the ears and tonsils. Tubal discharge (ears)
Nat Mur	White-coated tongue	This remedy can be summed up with three words: Malnutrition, dehydrated and weak. Worse being consoled, worse 10am, worse when at the ocean, loss of vital fluids will cause symptoms, discharge is clear and in large quantities, craves salt, eczema in the creases of joints/forehead/edge of scalp, herpetic rashes especially after illness, dry and cracked skin, chapped lips
Merc Sol	Canker sores, profuse saliva, tongue is moist and coated	This remedy has an affinity for the digestive and renal systems with specific action on throat. Foul-smelling breath, gums are white/yellow color and ulcers in gums, tooth abscess, sores in mouth, intense thirst, thick tongue, salivate heavily, parotiditis, heavy perspiration especially at night and offensive in odor, ulcers, worse at night, known as "the human thermometer," shivering and goose-bumps
Sul Ac	Patches in gum and on tongue	This remedy is for severe weakness. Worse from cold and smell of coffee, better from heat, internal trembling, hemorrhaging black blood
Thuja	White-coated tongue	This remedy has an affinity for the skin, mucus, and any type of growths appearing inside of body or outside on the skin: warts, moles, acne, seborrhea,

		cradle cap, hair loss, scalp has white scaly dandruff Worse cold/humid weather/3 am or 3 pm, better with heat, discharges have a moldy smell

TONSILITIS

REMEDIES:

Apis, Belladonna, Ferrum Phos., Guaiacum, Hepar Sulph., Kali Mur, Mercurius Sol., Phytolacca

Remedy	Symptom Differentiation	Keynote Differentiation
Apis		This remedy is known for swelling, burning pain, and jealousy. Worse from heat, better from cold, hot dry skin, inflammation
Bell	Tonsils are scarlet red, burning pain, desire to swallow but hurts, constriction in throat, desires lemonade	Symptoms usually have sudden and violent onset, local congestion of blood (example face is red), the congested area is usually hot, children usually convulse when they have a fever
Ferr Phos	Acute tonsillitis, throat is red/burning/swollen, worse on waking up, difficulty swallowing, better with cold, hoarseness, over-use of voice	Tired, anemic, pale. Bleeds easily, low temperature, rapid pulse, face is red and pale alternatingly, hemorrhages easily, better with slow motion, craves sour things
Hep Sul	Tonsils are enlarged/throbbing/painful, swallowing painful, radiates to ears	This remedy is hypersensitive especially to touch and cold air, worse dry/cold weather/slightest draft, better with heat, craves sour things especially vinegar
Merc Sol	Tonsils are swollen, pain radiates to ear, ulcerated, worse on right side	This remedy has an affinity for the digestive and renal systems with specific action on throat. Foul-smelling breath, gums are white/yellow color and ulcers

		in gums, tooth abscess, sores in mouth, intense thirst, thick tongue, salivate heavily, parotiditis, heavy perspiration especially at night and offensive in odor, ulcers, worse at night, known as "the human thermometer," shivering and goose-bumps
Phyt	Swollen tonsils	This remedy has an affinity for the mucus, breasts and bones. Worse with cold/wet/motion, better with dry weather and resting. Stiffness and bruising all over body, sciatica

TRAVEL PROBLEMS

REMEDIES:

Arsenicum Album, Cocculus, Petroleum, Tabacum

Remedy	Symptom Differentiation	Keynote Differentiation
Ars	Traveler's Diarrhea	This remedy has an affinity for mucus, kidneys liver, adrenal glands and the nervous system. This remedy can be summed up in three words: weak, restless and cold (temperature-wise). Burning pains, worse 1-3am and from the cold, thirsty for small amounts of cold water, fear of death, food-poisoning
Cocc	Jetlag, Motion-sickness	# 1 Jetlag remedy. This remedy has an affinity for treating spasms. Insomnia (especially from being a care-giver/mom), sadness, paralysis of facial nerve, worse from food/loss of sleep/open air/smoking/riding/ swimming/touch/drink/tobacco, trembling
Petro	Motion-sickness especially	This remedy has an affinity for

		sea-sickness	the skin and digestive mucus. Seasickness, worse from cold/winter/motion sickness, better in summer and heat, motion sickness better closing eyes, hands chapped (especially in winter), intense hunger and thirst, diarrhea only in morning
Tab		Motion-sickness especially sea-sickness	Nausea, vomiting, cold sweats, antiseptic properties, cholera-like symptoms, angina, constriction of throat/chest/bladder/rectum, vertigo

URINARY TRACT INFECTIONS

REMEDIES:

Apis, Aconite, Berberis, Cantharis, Mercurius Sol., Nux Vomica, Pulsatilla, Sarsparilla, Staphysagria

Remedy	Symptom Differentiation	Keynote Differentiation
Apis	Stinging, burning, worse at night and warmth, intense urge to urinate, urinates in drops	This remedy is known for swelling, burning pain, and jealousy. Worse from heat, better from cold, hot dry skin, inflammation
Acon	Early stages of UTI, painful urination, hot feeling during urination	This remedy has an affinity for the circulatory and nervous system. Worse extreme or sudden cold/extreme heat/night, better with perspiration, rapid pulse, sudden high fever, red skin, intense thirst for large quantities of cold water, restlessness, anxiety, fear of death, croup cough
Berb	Pain is burning/shooting/radiating to back/legs/abdomen/pelvis, bladder aches, worse with movement	Changeable symptoms: thirsty then thirstless, hungry then no appetite, gout, feels like a cap is over head, nausea before breakfast, thick and red urine, neuralgia under finger nails,

		worse from motion/standing/scratching
Canth	Burning pain, decreased urine flow, restlessness	This remedy has an affinity for the urinary tract and the skin. Pain is sharp (causes crying)/violent/piercing/burning in bladder, tendency to gangrene, feel like being "roasted alive" (intensity of burning pain), cystitis
Merc Sol	Strong urge to urinate, burning, chills, sweating, worse at night	This remedy has an affinity for the digestive and renal systems with specific action on throat. Foul-smelling breath, gums are white/yellow color and ulcers in gums, tooth abscess, sores in mouth, intense thirst, thick tongue, salivate heavily, parotiditis, heavy perspiration especially at night and offensive in odor, ulcers, worse at night, known as "the human thermometer," shivering and goose-bumps
Nux Vom	Constant urge to urinate, feels like needles, urge to pass stools, better from urinating and warm bath, worse from over-eating	This remedy as an affinity for the nervous and digestive system. Irritable, cold, hypersensitive, angry, worse after eating, better with sleep, tongue is yellow/white color, craves spicy and sour food, constipation, sneezing upon waking
Puls	UTI from sudden chill during hot weather, urgent desire to urinate, very emotional	This remedy has an affinity for the venous system and mucus. Changeable behavior, worse from heat, better from cold open air, thirstless, thick yellow/yellow-greenish discharge, worse after sunset
Sars	Girls need to stand to urinate, severe pain at the end of urination	This remedy has an affinity for the skin and mucus. Dry/shriveled/creased skin, purple and blue spots on skin,

		pain after urinating, unable to urinate while sitting-must stand, intense pain in kidneys especially right kidney
Staph	Urgent desire to urinate, feels like single drop still left	This remedy has an affinity for the urinary and genital system as well as the skin. Hypersensitive to emotions, excitable, irritated easily, obsessed about sexual ideas, burning/frequent/dripping urination, eczema with severe itching, styes especially on upper eyelids

VACCINATION SIDE EFFECTS

REMEDIES:

Hypericum, Ledum, Mezereum, Silica, Thuja

Remedy	Symptom Differentiation	Keynote Differentiation
Hyp	Acute reaction to vaccine	This remedy has an affinity for the nervous system, painful scars, worse after having tooth pulled
Led	Acute reaction to vaccine	This remedy has an affinity for the joints and the skin. Rheumatism, poison-ivy-like rash, tetanus, twitching, better from cold, worse at night and from heat of bed
Mez	Skin rash after vaccinations	This remedy has an affinity for the bones and the skin. Joints feel bruised and stiff, skin problems after vaccines, very sensitive to cold air, crusts on head look like leather, facial neuralgia, worse from cold air/night/until midnight/warm food/touch/motion, better from open air
Sil	MMR, DPT vaccine, red and	This remedy has an affinity for

	inflamed at site, convulsions, diarrhea, fever, abscess, nausea, asthma and backache since vaccine	the nervous system and is very malnourished. They are weak and demineralized. Worse cold and humid weather, better with heat, slinters (will push them out), fontanels stay open, perspire on head, abscess remedy, white spots on nails, weak nails/hair
Thuja	Asthma/cough/sleeplessness after vaccine	This remedy has an affinity for the skin, mucus, and any type of growths appearing inside of body or outside on the skin: warts, moles, acne, seborrhea, cradle cap, hair loss, scalp has white scaly dandruff Worse cold/humid weather/3 am or 3 pm, better with heat, discharges have a moldy smell

WEIGHT PROBLEMS

REMEDIES:

Baryta Carb., Calcarea Carb., Calcarea Phos., Magnesia Carb., Silica

Remedy	Symptom Differentiation	Keynote Differentiation
Bar Carb	Poor weight gain	This remedy has an affinity for the mental development, arteries, and lymphatic system. Late development/milestones, shy, worse cold/humid/thinking about problems
Calc Carb	Easy weight gain, early weight gain	Any Calcarea remedy has an affinity for bones, lymph nodes, circulation and polyps. They sweat profusely on head, babies teethe late, walk slow and are lazy, large appetite, remember the four F's: fat, fair skin, fainting, and fearful. If Ruta and Rhus Tox have stopped

		working, this remedy can be thought of. For chronic indications of pulsatilla
Calc Phos	Poor weight gain	This remedy has an affinity for the bones, blood, lymph nodes and works on the nutrition of the body. Teeth are long, narrow and yellow, bones are long and straight, tired and nervous, rickets, weight loss, repetitive sore throat/bronchitis/colds
Mag Carb	Poor weight gain	This remedy has an affinity for the digestive tract, female genitals, and nervous system. Very sensitive to cold, worse from resting and temperature change, better moving around and walking outside, acute shooting pains along the nerves
Sil	Poor weight gain	This remedy has an affinity for the nervous system and is very malnourished. They are weak and demineralized. Worse cold and humid weather, better with heat, slinters (will push them out), fontanels stay open, perspire on head, abscess remedy, white spots on nails, weak nails/hair

WHOOPING COUGH

REMEDIES:

Antimonium Tart., Carbo Veg., Cuprum, Drosera, Kali Sulph., Phosphorus, Sanguinaria Canadensis

Remedy	Symptom Differentiation	Keynote Differentiation
Ant Tart	Breathing is asthmatic/difficult/fast/rattling/loud, vomiting with or after cough, whooping	This remedy has an affinity for the respiratory

	cough, difficult to bring up mucus, sleepy with cough	system and the skin. This remedy can be summed up with three words: exhaustion, paleness, and sleepiness. Spitting behavior, grasps for other people
Carbo Veg	Fast breathing and wheezing, cough is in fits/racking/suffocative/violent/whooping, mucus is green, dry heaving (retching), hoarseness, worse evening before midnight	This remedy has an affinity for the digestive system and the body's circulation. Lack of reaction, engorged veins, slow recovery of previous illness, sluggish, listless, indifferent
Cup	Breathing difficult and fast, cough is in long/uninterrupted/irregular fits/violent/whooping, worse from cold air, better from sips of cold water	This remedy has an affinity for the muscular system. Spasmodic pain begins and ends suddenly, convulsions, blue face, violent cramping, whooping cough, better drinking a sip of cold water, violent diarrhea with cramping pains
Dros	Cough is dry/quick/tearing/spasmodic/hacking/irritating/barking, tickling in larynx, wheezes when inhaling, whooping cough, breathing is difficult in between coughing fits, face turns blue from coughing, vomiting from	This remedy has an affinity for the mucus of the larynx and bronchi, as well as the lymphatic

	cough, mucus is bloody, nosebleeds from cough, abdominal pain from cough which is better with pressure, worse from drinking/lying down/talking/after midnight, fast and difficult breathing, pain in chest from cough, dry heaving (retching), cough from measles	system and bones. Worse at night/heat of bed/laughing/singing, better from moving
Kali Sul	Whooping and rattling cough, mucus is difficult to bring up/swallows it/yellow, worse at night/warm room/stuffy room/heat	This remedy has an affinity for the mucus and skin. Irritable, angry and obstinate, worse from heat/evening/resting, better from cold air/outdoors/walking, throbbing pains, bronchitis, asthma, eczema
Phos	Difficult breathing, cough is dry at night/tickling in larynx/irritating/racking/tight/violent, mucus is green/large amount/tastes sweet and salty/white/yellow, burning pain in chest from cough, sweating from cough, better sitting up, worse change of temperature/fever/reading aloud	This remedy is highly sensitive especially to light, noises, and smells. Fear of thunderstorm, worse from cold/storms/left side, better from sleep, craves salt and cold drinks, midnight "snacker" especially around 3 am, #1 morning sickness remedy
Sang	Cough is dry/spasmodic/raw, worse at night and cold room, mucus is burning, sneezing	This remedy has an affinity for the circulatory system and the mucus. Worse from

		sun/odors/every 7 days, better from sleep and passing gas

WORMS

REMEDIES:

Calcarea Carb., Cina, Silica

Remedy	Symptom Differentiation	Keynote Differentiation
Calc Carb	Tapeworm	Any Calcarea remedy has an affinity for bones, lymph nodes, circulation and polyps. They sweat profusely on head, babies teethe late, walk slow and are lazy, large appetite, remember the four F's: fat, fair skin, fainting, and fearful. If Ruta and Rhus Tox have stopped working, this remedy can be thought of. For chronic indications of pulsatilla
Cina	Itching from worms	Convulsions beginning on one side of the face, attack stops and begins at the same time, breathing slows down, urine incontinence, do not like to be touched or looked at, large circles under the eyes, sickly appearance, yawn frequently, grinding of teeth, restless sleep, frequent rubbing of nose and scratching of nostrils, constant hunger that is not easily satiable, pain in belly-button better by lying on abdomen, worse during new moon and full moon, better lying on stomach/abdomen, presence of round worms, teething

Sil	Worms during teething	This remedy has an affinity for the nervous system and is very malnourished. They are weak and demineralized. Worse cold and humid weather, better with heat, slinters (will push them out), fontanels stay open, perspire on head, abscess remedy, white spots on nails, weak nails/hair

REFERENCES

Boericke, William MD. *Homeopathic Materia Medica.* Reprint. Santa Rosa, CA: Boericke & Tafel 1927

Castro, Miranda. *Homeopathy for Pregnancy, Birth, and Your Baby's First Year.* New York: St. Martin's 1993

Hahnemann, Samuel. *Organon of Medicine.* Reprint. New Delhi: B. Jain.

Jouanny, Jacques, MD. *The Essentials of Homeopathic Materia Medica.* France: Boiron 1984

Murphy, Robin. *Homeopathic Clinical Repertory: A Modern, Alphabetical and Practical Repertory.* Virginia: Lotus Health 2005

Schmidt, Michael A. *Childhood Ear Infections: What Every Parent and Physician Should Know About Prevention, Home Care, and Alternative Treatment.* California: North Atlantic Books 1990

Ullman, Dana. *Homeopathic Medicine for Children and Infants.* New York: G.P. Putnam's Sons 1992

Made in the USA
Charleston, SC
11 November 2013